How to Deal with Menstrual Cramps

Natural Remedies to Stop Period Pains Without Medication

By

Erika Robinson

Table of Contents

Introduction

A lot of women experience serious pains and cramps during menstruation. The medical name for painful menstruation is called "Dysmenorrhea," and it is also called "menstrual cramps."

This throbbing and cramping pain occurs in the lower abdomen, thighs, and back and it comes along with uncomfortable signs and symptoms like nausea, vomiting, diarrhea, headaches, moodiness, irritability, and fatigue.

Menstrual cramps can be treated, and the treatment depends on the types and causes. In severe menstrual cramps like that of secondary dysmenorrhea, surgical methods of treatment can be used.

Possible Causes of Menstrual Cramps
There are two main types of period pains, and each has different causes-- they are primary and secondary dysmenorrhea.

Primary dysmenorrhea is the most common type of menstrual cramps, and it is not caused by an underlying medical condition. Secondary dysmenorrhea is instigated by another condition (underlying medical condition) and it usually occurs later in life.

Primary dysmenorrhea is caused mainly excess amount of prostaglandins in the body. This is a hormone made by the uterus, and it makes the muscles of the womb to relax and tighten-- this is the main cause of primary cramps.

During your menstrual cycle, your uterus (womb) contracts and it contracts more when you are menstruating. When this happens, it presses the blood vessels thereby preventing the supply of oxygen to the muscles and tissues of the womb.

The pain experienced comes from the inability of the womb to get sufficient oxygen.

Secondary dysmenorrhea is caused by a medical condition affecting the womb and reproductive system. Examples of these conditions are uterine fibroids, infections, adenomyosis, and endometriosis.

This starts later in life and not when you are younger as in primary dysmenorrhea.

Causes of Primary Menstrual Cramps

Primary dysmenorrhea can be triggered or aggravated by some factors such as:

- Stress
- Insufficient sleep
- Unhealthy diet
- High intake of alcohol
- Smoking
- Obesity
- High intake of salt and sugar
- Inadequate intake of water or dehydration
- Negative emotions and thoughts
- Sedentary lifestyle

It also gets worse as time goes on. Menstrual cramps start one or two days before the period and last for a few days, especially in primary dysmenorrhea. In secondary dysmenorrhea, the pain can continue even after your menstruation has stopped.

Also, secondary menstrual pains begin quite earlier than primary pains. It also lasts longer, and does not come along with menstrual pain symptoms like diarrhea, nausea, vomiting, and fatigue.

Primary menstrual cramps usually get less painful as you age or when you give birth. It even stops completely after childbirth for some women.

Causes of Secondary Menstrual Cramps

Diseases affecting the reproductive organs are responsible for secondary dysmenorrhea, and some of these diseases are:

- Uterine Fibroids: These are growth found on the inner walls of your womb. The major signs of uterine fibroids are agonizing pains and a heavy flow.

- Dislodged Intrauterine Device (IUD): This can lead to menstrual cramps, although some cramps are noticed after implantation. This is quite normal and one of the side effects of IUD.

However, if the pain is so severe and lasts up to several days after implantation, you have to see a gynecologist as soon as possible. He/she will carry out a pelvic exam to see if the strings are coming out of the cervix and adjust it if so.

- Pelvic Inflammatory Disease: This is a bacterial infection that starts in the womb and spreads to other reproductive organs. This condition is characterized by consistent dull pain and vaginal discharge.

Untreated STDs like gonorrhea and chlamydia can cause a serious infection of the fallopian tubes, ovaries, and uterus, thereby causing this infection.

- Endometriosis: In this condition, the tissues which line the uterus get inflamed. At times, the tissues are found outside the uterus. It also develops on other organs such as the fallopian tubes.

  10% of women going through dysmenorrhea are affected by endometriosis. When you have this condition, medications and painkillers may not work for pains.

- Cervical Stenosis: It occurs when the opening to your uterus becomes narrow.

- Ectopic pregnancy or miscarriage: This condition happens when the fertilization occurs elsewhere other than the uterus. Places such as the fallopian tubes. Fertilization won't take place, and it will cause severe bleeding and pains.

- Adenomyosis: It occurs when the tissues lining the uterus grows and expands into the muscles of the womb.

- Ovarian cysts: In this condition, a cyst or many cysts may rupture the ovaries, making it twist and have a reduced flow of blood.

This condition is characterized by a sharp and stabbing pain that occurs on one side of the body. It can also be accompanied by nausea and vomiting.

How to Diagnose the Cause of Period Pains

A pelvic exam can help your doctor know the exact cause of menstrual cramps, especially for severe cases. They might also carry out imaging tests like ultrasound on you to diagnose the condition properly.

If your doctor is suspecting it to be a Secondary Dysmenorrhea, he will have you go through a laparoscopy—a surgical procedure that helps doctors look inside your body to see what's wrong.

Natural Home Remedies to Relieve Menstrual Cramps

There are lots of effective natural remedies that can stop and prevent menstrual cramps, some are even more effective than these painkiller medications, and they also don't have side effects except combined with certain drugs.

In this book are some of the most effective natural therapies for menstrual cramps. Please check with a doctor or naturopath before trying any of these if you are on medication to prevent drug-herb interaction.

Ginger and garlic shouldn't be taken if you are on hypertension and cholesterol medications.

1. Healthy Diet

Intake of bad and unhealthy foods can increase menstrual cramps because they cause nutritional deficiencies. There are some nutrients which control inflammation and help the body manage pains; example is magnesium.

Your diet is one of the keys to painless menstruation. Avoid processed, preserved, and sugary foods. The right kind of food will relieve pain and inflammation, during your period, eat lots of anti-inflammatory foods like tomatoes, cherries, bell pepper, squash, and blueberries.

Increase your intake of fruits, vegetables, healthy fats, herbs, and water. This will help to prevent or reduce period pains to an extent. A study involving 33 women with menstrual pains showed that they had less pains when they took a low-fat vegetarian diet.

Another study showed that women who took organic dairy had less menstrual pains than women who took none. This is accredited to the presence of calcium and vitamin D.

Coldwater fish is rich in omega-3 fatty acids-- this nutrient calms inflammation and improves menstrual cramps. Eat calcium-rich foods like dark green vegetables, almonds, and beans because this mineral helps fight inflammation.

Magnesium is another powerful nutrient needed by women, its deficiency in the body leads to increased menstrual cramps, and it also causes stress, anxiety, and body pains.

More than 30 enzymes in your body depend on magnesium; it is also required for the proper functioning of the muscles, nerves, and heart. When taken along with vitamin B6, magnesium relieves the symptoms of menstrual cramps.

Don't take magnesium supplements if you are on some medications like antibiotics, bisphosphonates, diuretics, and proton pump inhibitors.

Moderate intake of magnesium helps in reducing the risks of endometriosis, a cause of secondary dysmenorrhea. Natural foods containing magnesium are black beans, peanuts, cashews, spinach, and almonds.

Calcium-rich foods and calcium supplements help relieve menstrual cramps because they act on your nervous system, muscles, and heart. Adequate consumption of this vital nutrient will lessen menstrual cramps.

2. Increase Your Water Intake

Dehydration and insufficient intake of water increase the symptoms of menstrual cramps and make it worse. It relieves bloating, headaches, mood swings, and sleepiness.

Drink up to 8 glasses of water daily. You can also include other healthy fluids like lemon water, herbal teas like ginger or Moringa tea, unsweetened homemade fruit juices, smoothies, and fruits and vegetables.

Avoid alcohol and carbonated drinks-- they increase dehydration and aggravate menstrual cramps. So, avoid these when you are on your period or about seeing your period.

Women who vomit and experience diarrhea during their period should replace lost fluids by drinking plenty of water.

3. Ginger

This is one of the most active natural painkillers, and it also has a strong anti-inflammatory effect. It is a safe and effective home remedy for menstrual cramps if you are not on blood pressure medications.

Ginger root is even more effective than some painkillers, and it has no side effects. It works by reducing the levels of prostaglandins. It dismisses exhaustion and fights irregular menstruation.

Drink warm ginger tea when on your period and if you have severe pain, start drinking it a few days to your period. You can also use warm ginger water as a compress-- place it on your abdomen for pain relief.

Add black pepper or turmeric to your ginger tea, to make it more effective.

4. Fennel

Fennel herbal teas and supplements help in relieving menstrual cramps and symptoms. It stops uterine contractions, a powerful pain reliever, and it is particularly beneficial to women who have severe menstrual pain and can't go about their normal duties.

5. Pycnogenol Extract

This is a plant extract derived from pine trees found in the southwest region of France. It contains lots of antioxidants which help in relieving dysmenorrhea and its symptoms.

This herb is so effective in relieving cramps. In a study, women between the ages of 18 to 48 years old were given 60 mg of Pycnogenol extract during their periods. Observations have found that the pains reduced significantly, and they can thrive without painkillers.

Even after the women stopped taking this extract, they still had less need for pain medications. You can find this in a good health store, or a reputable online store.

6. Turmeric

Curcumin, the powerful active ingredient in turmeric is a strong pain reliever. When taken 7 days before menstruation, it relieves the symptoms of painful menstruation and even PMS as well.

Curcumin also fights inflammation, and it changes the levels of the neurotransmitter, thereby helping in relieving the symptoms of menstrual cramps and PMS.

Take turmeric tea or turmeric capsules days before your period begin and continue till three days after your period.

7. Heat

The heat helps in relaxing the muscles of the uterus and has been used as an effective way to relieve menstrual cramps. You can make use of heating pads which you can purchase from any health store, or you can even make yours at home.

Soak a clean cloth or towel in hot-warm water and squeeze lightly. Put the towel in another cloth and place it on your abdomen. You can also put hot water in a bottle and place it on your abdomen.

Try taking your bath with Epsom salt. Some people have found relief from their cramps with this method. Mix the warm water with Epsom salt and soak in it for 20 minutes or have your bath with it.

This heat therapy also works from inside-- you can drink hot liquids like teas, soups, or warm water. This will help to relax your internal muscles.

8. Vitamin D

Studies show that little quantities of vitamin D in the body leads to increased production of prostaglandins in the body. These chemicals make the womb to contract, leading to menstrual cramps.

Also, when there are present in your bloodstream, it leads to nausea, vomiting, and diarrhea. Increase your intake of vitamin D to reduce the rate at which your body produces prostaglandins.

Vitamin D also helps in treating pains, including menstrual pains. Expose yourself to moderate sunlight for at least 20 minutes daily. Also, increase your intake of eggs-- they are one of the best dietary sources of vitamin D.

You can meet a doctor to prescribe a good vitamin D supplement for you.

9. Avoid Caffeine

Some women have found relief from period cramps just by eliminating caffeine from their diet. Caffeine is present in many drinks, like energy drinks, chocolate, soda, tea, and coffee.

If you are addicted to caffeine, then you need to reduce your intake slowly so that you can stop successfully without any withdrawal symptom.

Healthier alternatives to caffeine are dark leafy greens, proteins, berries, and vegetable smoothies. They give you a high level of energy, and there are no side effects like in the case of caffeine intake.

10. Massage

Massage is a powerful relief for menstrual cramps, and you can lessen the pain just by massaging your abdomen for 5 minutes. It increases the flow of blood to your organs, and it relieves the symptoms of dysmenorrhea.

You can make the massage more effective, like using essential oils like ginger essential oil, marjoram, clary sage, and lavender essential oils. Mix them with a carrier oil like olive oil, jojoba oil, or coconut oil before applying it directly on your skin.

It prevents skin reactions, especially in people with sensitive and delicate skins.

11. Have Quality Sleep

Poor sleep can affect your health in many ways, and menstrual cramps are one of them. Insomnia and short hours of sleep increase the pains of dysmenorrhea and its symptoms.

Quality sleep keeps menstrual cramps at bay. Have a healthy sleep routine and stick to it. As an adult, you shouldn't be sleeping for less than eight hours every night.

Avoid your TV, computer, and smartphone an hour before going to bed. Try new sleeping positions to know the one you are comfortable with.

Take dinner earlier, like an hour before going to bed. Additionally, drink a warm herbal tea like ginger tea, take a warm bath, and listen to soothing music before going to bed.

These will help promote healthy sleep and relieve the pains and symptoms of dysmenorrhea.

12. Essential Oils

These oils are gotten from medicinal plants, and they contain the active healing ingredients of those herbs in very high concentrations. That is why they have to be used with care and in little amounts to prevent toxicity.

There are a lot of essential oils that can help dismiss menstrual cramps, including PMS. Some of these oils can even be of great help for severe dysmenorrhea, and sometimes combining these oils make the therapy more effective.

Some essential oils cannot be used without a carrier oil, especially when you are applying it topically on your skin. These carrier oils help dilute the concentration of this highly powerful and concentrated oils, and they also carry the essential oils deep into your skin.

Examples of good carrier oils are coconut oil, olive oil, jojoba, and almond oil.

Some of the most effective essential oils for menstrual cramps are:

- Marjoram essential oil: This reduces pain and inflammation by reducing muscle spasms, and it also treats infections because it has a prevailing antibacterial property. Mix it with a carrier oil and use this blend to massage your abdomen and other body parts that might be paining you.
- Lavender essential oils: This oil has a lot of immense health benefits,

including fighting pains and sleeplessness. It is an excellent home remedy for menstrual cramps, you can massage your skin directly with this oil without mixing it with a carrier oil, or you can inhale it.

- Clary sage essential oil: This oil helps relieve the symptoms of menstrual cramps like moodiness, cramping, and it also induces peace of mind. It fights acne, one of the major symptoms of menstruation, because it has a strong antiseptic property. Massage your abdomen with this oil.

- Eucalyptus oil: This is one of the most common essential oils sold worldwide, it has a lot of benefits, and it is used in making a lot of products, including insect repellant and antiseptic.

  It has powerful anti-inflammatory properties. It boosts your immune system and lessens the severity of period cramps and symptoms. Rub this oil on your abdomen and massage it softly.

- Rose essential oil: This oil relieves cramps and other symptoms of menstrual cramps, and it also treats irregular period. It makes your cycle normal and balances the levels of hormones.

Rosemary oil promotes the health of your uterus, and it fights depression and mood swings during menstruation. You can inhale it or apply it topically on your abdomen and massage it.

- Tea tree oil: This oil is specifically active against pimples and breakouts before and during menstruation, and it also clears spots caused by those breakouts. You have to dilute this oil with a carrier oil of your choice before applying it on your face. You can use a face cream containing tea tree essential oil to prevent or manage breakouts during periods.

- Ylang ylang essential oil: This oil has a lot of benefits for women suffering from dysmenorrhea. It boosts mood and fight moodiness. It is also a powerful natural antiseptic, thus fighting the bacteria responsible for acne.
  Inhale it or mix it with a carrier oil and massage your abdomen with the mixture to relieve cramps. You can also rub the mixture on your face to control pimples and outbreaks.
- Peppermint essential oil: Peppermint oil relieve fatigue, mood swings, and sleeplessness during menstruation. It also controls your appetite, thus

stopping those cravings for sugar and salts which can worsen the condition.

It is energizing, so inhaling it is enough to give you all these benefits.

- Neroli essential oil: This oil is gotten from the blossoms of the orange tree. It has a strong relaxing and stress-relieving properties. It balances the levels of hormones and fights anxiety and stress. Inhale this oil to relieve the symptoms of menstrual cramps.

- Orange essential oil: orange oil and other oils gotten from citrus fruits relax the body and improve your mood. Inhale this oil to reap its immense benefits.

13. Acupuncture

This is an eastern method of healing used all around the world. Acupuncture and acupressure stimulate unique trigger points on the skin to produce the desired effect on your body.

A well-trained acupuncturist can use needles to reduce your menstrual cramps. These therapies are also very effective for many health conditions, including strokes.

The acupuncturist knows where these trigger points are, and he/she knows how to trigger them using pressure. In the case of acupressure, the pressure is applied to key areas of your body like the abdomen, back, feet, thumb, and index finger to relief pains.

These therapies are drug-free, and they can be used any time, especially when the symptoms arise. You can also ask the therapist to show you how to do it yourself.

14. Avoid Salty Foods

Salts make you dehydrated, and dehydration worsens menstrual cramps. Avoid processed foods when you are on your period or about seeing your period because they contain a lot of salt.

15. Exercise

Exercise has helped many women find relief from menstrual cramps. It releases endorphins into your body-- this neurotransmitter gives a general feeling of happiness and well-being.

Exercises you can participate in during your period are running, walking, and other moderate exercises you can think off. Don't do any exercise that will get you tired or stressed out because fatigue is already a symptom of menstrual cramps.

Strenuous exercises can worsen fatigue.

16. Chinese Herbal Medicine

Chinese traditional medicine has been in existence for over 5,000 years, and till date, it is used to treat a lot of chronic diseases that conventional medicine can't.

Chinese herbal medicine is very effective in treating dysmenorrhea. According to studies, over 25% of women who couldn't get help from conventional medicine got it through Chinese therapy.

It relieved their pains and cleared all the symptoms of dysmenorrhea. Those who take Chinese herbs depend less on medications or don't even take them at all.

17. Vitamin B1 and Fish Oil

This combination is very effective for dysmenorrhea. It lessens the pain of menstruation and also shortens the duration of the pain. In the study that proved this, the women were given 100 mg of vitamin B1 and 500 mg of fish oil daily.

18. Dill

Studies have shown that dill is as effective and, in some cases, more effective than OTC painkillers. It is an effective non-drug remedy for menstrual cramps.

Dill capsules can be found in health shops, and if you have access to the leaves, you can boil it and take it as tea.

19. Cinnamon

Cinnamon is another powerful natural pain reliever. It relieves menstrual cramps, reduces bleeding, and also relieve the symptoms of period cramps such as nausea and vomiting.

It has no side effects, and you can take cinnamon herbal tea using the leaves or seeds. Alternatively, cinnamon pills or supplements are used. You can find them in a good health store.

Sprinkle cinnamon powder on your meals and drinks. Increase your intake of cinnamon before and during menstrual period, and you will have relief from pains.

20. Chamomile

Chamomile herbal tea reduces menstrual cramps and symptoms. It contains many anti-inflammatory substances that stop the effects of prostaglandins.

Aside from stopping menstrual cramps, chamomile tea also eases the flow of blood while you are menstruating.

21. Warm Baths

Warm baths relief pain, relax the nerves, muscles and also soothe the body. Make sure the water is not hot to avoid burning your skin. Add some drops of pain-relieving essential oils of your choice, and soak in this for at least 20 minutes.

Do this in the evenings more, and you will feel better and sleep better. If you don't have the facilities to soak, a warm shower has the same effect. It will lessen pelvic pain and other symptoms of dysmenorrhea.

22. Mint

These are beneficial in treating a lot of conditions like nausea, vomiting, stomach ache, and indigestion. Drink mint tea before and during your period, and it will relieve these pains.

23. Holy Basil

This is one of the most used healing herbs used in Ayurveda (Indian Traditional) medicine. It contains a high amount of a powerful painkiller called Eugenol. This makes it one of the best home remedies for menstrual cramps.

Boil the leaves and drink the decoction. You can also use it in preparing your meals.

24. Coriander

This is a powerful home remedy for dysmenorrhea, ancient Ayurvedic practitioners mentioned and used this herb in treating menstrual cramps and other menstrual problems.

Get a few fresh stems of coriander and boil it in a cup of water, drink this to relieve cramps and other symptoms of painful menstruation.

25. Asafetida

This is a powerful Indian herb used in treating menstrual cramps. It works by balancing the levels of your hormones, especially progesterone. It increases the amount of progesterone in your body, thus fighting uterine contractions and cramps.

26. CBD Oil

This is a powerful remedy for pains and inflammation, make sure you get it from a good and reputable health store and take it according to prescriptions.

27. Cumin Seeds

This herbal remedy has an anti-spasmodic effect; it even fights inflammation and relieves menstrual pains and cramps. Take cumin seed herbal tea daily when on your period to relieve the pains.

28. Beet Root

This amazing herb with a unique earthy taste is effective in correcting menstrual disorders and problems. Take a glass of beetroot daily when on your period.

29. Angelica Sinensis

This is a popular Chinese herb used in treating a lot of menstrual problems and disorders such as dysmenorrhea. It fights pain, relieves inflammation, and controls heavy bleeding.

You can get the tea bags from a good health shop. Take it according to the prescription on the pack.

30. Parsley

This wonderful herb can regulate your cycle, thus fighting irregular cycle and other menstrual disorders. It fights cramps and regulate bleeding. Boil the leaves and take it as tea or you can combine it with other vegetables like cucumbers, beetroots, tomatoes, and carrots. Blend it and take it as smoothie before and during your period.

31. Orgasm

There are quite a handful of reports that orgasms help relieve menstrual cramps.

The uterus is relaxed before orgasm, and when you climax, the flow of blood to your uterus increases, thereby relieving the cramps.

Orgasms also release endorphins; the "feel good" messengers of the body, this, in turn, relieves pains, relaxes you, and help you feel better. They also induce sleep and relieve stress.

32. Green Tea

This popular drink is rich in catechins; this group of flavonoids has analgesic and antioxidant properties. It is one of the most widely used home therapies for menstrual cramps.

Add the green tea leaves or tea bags to a cup of water and boil it, leave it for 5 minutes to simmer and then you strain it, leave it to get warm before drinking it.

Make sure you drink it warm so that the heat can increase the effectiveness. Do this thrice daily when on your period.

33. Kinesiology Tape

Kinesiology tape is not for athletes only, anybody can use it. It helps relieve pains, aches, and cramps by increasing the circulation of blood and range of motion.

When you are having menstrual pains, put this tape around your pelvis, it will relieve the tension in that area, thereby reducing menstrual cramps.

Tie the tapes vertically and horizontally around your pelvic area, and make sure you focus more on where you have the pain. Go to a sports shop and ask for this tape-- cut off 2 pieces to convenience.

34. Transcutaneous nerve Stimulation

In this method of treating menstrual cramps, a small device is used to pass low-voltage electric current into the skin. This raises the pain threshold of the patient, and it stimulates your body to release endorphins, a hormone that makes you feel good and relieves pains.

This method can also be used along with other methods like medications, heat, and natural remedies.

35. Sesame Seeds

This is an effective Indian traditional remedy for dysmenorrhea; it is mostly used in treating menstrual cramps. You can chew on freshly boiled sesame seeds or mash it into a thick paste and eat it.

Sesame is a storehouse of linolenic acid; this compound is an antioxidant with strong anti-inflammatory properties. You can also massage your abdomen with sesame oil.

36. Fenugreek Seeds

Fenugreek seeds have high amounts of lysine and proteins rich in tryptophan, this is responsible for its medicinal properties, and it helps in treating menstrual cramps by reducing pains.

Soak some teaspoons of fenugreek seeds inside a cup of water and let it stay overnight or for 12 hours, then strain and drink the water before eating (on an empty stomach). Do this daily during your period, and you will have less or no pain.

37. Maca

Maca is a powerful herb that helps to balance the levels of hormones and increase libido, thus fighting menstrual cramps. It also increases the duration of sleep, thus fighting insomnia. Maca increases fertility and boosts your skin's health.

This herb is available in capsules and powder forms. The effects are cumulative; this means you have to take it regularly for 3 or 5 weeks before you can see positive results.

Pregnant women should not consume this herb in any form to prevent complications.

38. Dong Quai

This wonderful Chinese herb helps relieves pains. It is a powerful anti-spasmodic herb and one of the most potent natural remedies for menstrual cramps.

It is available in the form of capsules, tea, or liquid version in a good health store or pharmacy.

39. Aloe Vera Juice

This herb has powerful healing and anti-inflammatory effects; it improves the flow of blood to the uterus, thus relieving the pains or reducing its intensity.

Those who have severe pains should start drinking Aloe Vera juice a few days to their periods while those with mild to moderate pains can start taking it when their period starts. Do this daily until your period ends.

40. Pickle Juice

This rehydrates your body and fights dehydration, thereby relieving pains caused by dehydration. It is even effective for post-exercise cramps. Drink half a cup of pickle juice as soon as you start feeling pains but don't take it on an empty stomach.

Ensure you have eaten first before drinking pickle juice.

41. Bupleurum

This is another powerful Chinese herb used in treating menstrual cramps; it relieves depression, moodiness, and cramps. Take the capsules according to prescription.

42. Red Raspberry Leaf

This is a popular natural remedy known for fighting menstrual disorders and infertility; it also relieves Cramps and PMS. It contains a high amount of calcium, a powerful uterine tonic which helps prevent cramping.

The capsules are available in good health stores. If you have access to the leaves, you can boil it and drink the tea warm. This will help relieve your menstrual cramps.

43. Chasteberry

The fruit of this herb is highly effective in treating PMS and menstrual cramps and disorders. It balances the levels of hormones and also relieves symptoms of dysmenorrhea caused by uterine fibroids.

Chasteberry, also known as vitex, balances the levels of estrogen to progesterone and prevents fibroids from happening in the first place. It also reduces fibroids. Chasteberry is available in liquid form or tablets. You should follow the prescription.

Medical Options for Treating Menstrual Cramps
1. Painkillers

Doctors prescribe painkillers and NSAID like ibuprofen and aspirin to stop the inflammation and pains. These drugs reduce the effects of prostaglandins, thereby relieving the pains and making you feel comfortable.

Those with severe pains can take these drugs earlier on before their period arrives. This will reduce the pains drastically. These drugs don't work for some, but it is still a good way to start fighting the pains.

Also, these drugs also have unpleasant side effects, especially when taken continuously. Ensure you take them according to prescription.

2. Hormonal Birth Control Pills

Birth control pills work for menstrual cramps, and it shortens the bleeding days and the rate of bleeding, and also gives fewer cramps and pains. They work by regulating the functions of prostaglandins.

Other hormonal birth control methods work by preventing ovulation. Example is the *ring and the pill*. These, in turn, will prevent the uterus from creating a thick lining in the first place.

Hormonal IUD helps thin the thick lining in the uterus, and it leaves no lining for shedding. You can check with your doctor to know which hormonal contraceptive is good for you and also find out about the possible side effects.

3. Surgery

Surgical procedures are used in treating secondary dysmenorrhea like fibroids, endometriosis, and other reproductive system disorders. When the hidden cause is corrected, the symptoms vanish.

In some cases where other approaches have failed, the uterus will be removed completely, and you must have made up your mind not to have children before this is carried out.

When to Seek for Medical Help

Period pains are quite normal, but some signs shouldn't be taken for granted and you should seek help immediately if you notice any of the following:

- When painkillers and natural remedies don't work, and the pain is making it difficult for you to carry on with your daily activities or work
- When it is getting worse instead of getting better
- When you start having period cramps for the first time, especially when you are over 25
- When you fall sick or have a fever along with your period pain

- When you feel the pains even after your period has ended or when you are not having your period.

Conclusion

These natural remedies will help you relieve menstrual cramps, but you have to follow instructions and avoid combining two herbs. Do not take some herbs with drugs and ask your doctor if some supplements and herbal extracts go with the medication you are taking.

—